Low Glycemic Index Diet

A Beginner's Step-by-Step Guide with Recipes and a Meal Plan

mf

copyright © 2019 Bruce Ackerberg

All rights reserved No part of this book may be reproduced, or stored in a retrieval system, or transmitted in any form or by any means, electronic, mechanical, photocopying, recording, or otherwise, without express written permission of the publisher.

Disclaimer

By reading this disclaimer, you are accepting the terms of the disclaimer in full. If you disagree with this disclaimer, please do not read the guide.

All of the content within this guide is provided for informational and educational purposes only, and should not be accepted as independent medical or other professional advice. The author is not a doctor, physician, nurse, mental health provider, or registered nutritionist/dietician. Therefore, using and reading this guide does not establish any form of a physician-patient relationship.

Always consult with a physician or another qualified health provider with any issues or questions you might have regarding any sort of medical condition. Do not ever disregard any qualified professional medical advice or delay seeking that advice because of anything you have read in this guide. The information in this guide is not intended to be any sort of medical advice and should not be used in lieu of any medical advice by a licensed and qualified medical professional.

The information in this guide has been compiled from a variety of known sources. However, the author cannot attest to or guarantee the accuracy of each source and thus should not be held liable for any errors or omissions.

You acknowledge that the publisher of this guide will not be held liable for any loss or damage of any kind incurred as a result of this guide or the reliance on any information provided within this guide. You acknowledge and agree that you assume all risk and responsibility for any action you undertake in response to the information in this guide.

Using this guide does not guarantee any particular result (e.g., weight loss or a cure). By reading this guide, you acknowledge that there are no guarantees to any specific outcome or results you can expect.

All product names, diet plans, or names used in this guide are for identification purposes only and are the property of their respective owners. The use of these names does not imply endorsement. All other trademarks cited herein are the property of their respective owners.

Where applicable, this guide is not intended to be a substitute for the original work of this diet plan and is, at most, a supplement to the original work for this diet plan and never a direct substitute. This guide is a personal expression of the facts of that diet plan.

Where applicable, persons shown in the cover images are stock photography models and the publisher has obtained the rights to use the images through license agreements with third-party stock image companies.

Table of Contents

Disclaimer — 3
Table of Contents — 5
Introduction — 6
Chapter 1: Carbohydrates and the Glycemic Index — 8
   Understanding Carbohydrates — 8
   The Glycemic Index (GI) — 8
   The Glycemic Load Rating — 10
Chapter 2: Low Glycemic Index Diet — 12
   Principles of the Low GI Diet — 12
   Benefits of Low Glycemic Index Diet — 14
   Disadvantages of a Low Glycemic Diet — 15
   Foods to Eat — 16
   Foods to Avoid — 17
Chapter 3: Week 1: Getting Started — 19
   List down your current diet / current food list — 19
   Find alternative food for high-value numbers — 21
   Finalizing your list — 22
Chapter 4: Week 2: Creating Your Meal Plan — 24
   Creating your recipes — 24
   Creating Your Meal Plan — 27
   Day 1 — 28
   Day 2 — 29
   Day 3 — 30
   Day 4 — 31
   Day 5 — 32
Chapter 5: Sample Recipes — 34
   Crab Stuffed Avocados — 34
   Beef Stew — 35
   Lemon Chicken Salad — 36

Grilled Tenderloin	37
Quinoa and Black Beans	38
Braised Balsamic Chicken	40
Tomato and Basil Soup	41
Lean Roast Beef Sandwich on Barley Bread	42
Beef and Mushroom Pie	43
Grilled Lamb	45
Buckwheat Pancakes with Blueberries	46
Almond Butter Banana Smoothie	47
Grilled Eggplant and Zucchini Salad	48
Sweet Potato and Black Bean Tacos	49
Chickpea and Kale Curry	50
Chapter 6: Week 3: Evaluation and Adjustments	**52**
Keeping a Record	52
Implementing Your Meal Plan	53
Making Necessary Adjustments	55
Evaluating Your Progress	56
Importance of Record Keeping	58
Planning Ahead	59
Chapter 7: The Last Step: Make it a Habit	**61**
Practical Tips for Sustaining a Low Glycemic Diet	61
Conclusion	**64**
FAQs	**66**
References and Helpful Links	**68**

Introduction

If you're struggling with maintaining consistent energy levels throughout your day or finding it challenging to manage a healthy weight, despite trying various diets, you might find some value in this guide. Here, we'll introduce the idea of the Low Glycemic Index (GI) Diet - an evidence-based approach to nutrition that may give you a fresh outlook on food.

The Low Glycemic Index Diet isn't about quick fixes but rather emphasizes lasting lifestyle changes that are rooted in scientific research. The idea behind it is quite straightforward: focus on consuming foods with a low GI value. These types of foods are digested and absorbed more slowly by your body, resulting in a gradual introduction of glucose into your bloodstream. This process is key because it helps keep your energy levels stable, reduces feelings of hunger, and potentially aids in weight management.

Imagine living a life where you don't constantly feel hungry or experience sudden dips in energy. Imagine enjoying a wide variety of tasty foods without having to worry about unexpected rises in your blood sugar levels. This can be more than just a hopeful aspiration - it can become a practical reality through the Low GI Diet.

In this guide, we will talk about the following;

- Carbohydrates and the Glycemic Index
- High vs Low GI Foods
- The Glycemic Load Rating
- Low Glycemic Index Diet
- Principles, Benefits, and Disadvantages of the Low GI Diet
- Foods To Eat and To Avoid
- Weekly Step Guide to Incorporate Low Glycemic Index Diet
- Sample Recipes and Meal Plan
- Practical Tips for Sustaining a Low Glycemic Diet

Keep reading as we break down the Low Glycemic Index Diet in this all-encompassing guide. We'll demystify the scientific principles behind it, highlight its many health benefits, suggest practical strategies for embracing it, and even introduce some delicious low GI recipes to kickstart your journey towards better health. So, gear up to absorb, learn, and navigate this compelling dietary exploration with us.

Chapter 1: Carbohydrates and the Glycemic Index

Before we get into Low Glycemic Diet, let's discuss what Low Glycemic Index is

Understanding Carbohydrates

Carbohydrates are one of the three main types of nutrients our bodies need to function properly, alongside proteins and fats. They serve as the body's primary source of energy. There are three main types of carbohydrates: sugars, starches, and fiber.

- **Sugars** are the simplest form of carbohydrates and include both naturally occurring sugars, like those in fruits and milk, and added sugars, like those in candies and sodas.
- **Starches** are complex carbohydrates that are made up of many sugar units bonded together. They are found in foods like grains, potatoes, and beans.
- **Fiber** is a type of carbohydrate that the body can't digest. It helps regulate the body's use of sugars, keeping hunger and blood sugar in check.

The Glycemic Index (GI)

The Glycemic Index (GI) is a ranking system for carbohydrates based on their impact on blood glucose levels.

It was developed to help people with diabetes manage their condition, but it's also used by people looking to lose weight or maintain a healthy weight.

Foods are ranked on a scale from 0 to 100, with pure glucose serving as the reference point (GI of 100). A food's GI value indicates how quickly it raises blood sugar levels after consumption:

- Low GI: 55 or less
- Medium GI: 56-69
- High GI: 70 or more

High vs Low GI Foods

High GI foods, such as white bread and potatoes, are rapidly digested and absorbed, leading to significant fluctuations in blood sugar levels. These rapid changes can lead to a cycle of high and low energy levels and stimulate feelings of hunger more quickly after eating.

Conversely, low-GI foods, like whole oats and most fruits and vegetables, are digested and absorbed more slowly, causing a slower, more sustained release of glucose into the bloodstream. This can help control appetite, delay hunger cues, and manage energy levels.

It's important to remember that while the GI can be a useful tool, it doesn't provide a complete picture of a food's nutritional value. It's also crucial to consider factors like portion size and the overall balance of a meal. A dietitian or healthcare professional can provide guidance on how to apply the principles of the GI in a balanced, healthy diet.

The Glycemic Load Rating

The Glycemic Load (GL) is a ranking system for the glycemic impact of foods, similar to the Glycemic Index (GI). However, while the GI only considers the quality of the carbohydrates in a food, the GL also takes into account the quantity of carbohydrates in a typical serving of that food.

Here's how it works: A food's Glycemic Load is calculated by multiplying its Glycemic Index by the amount of carbohydrates in one serving and then dividing by 100.

GL Ratings are classified as follows:

- Low: 10 or less
- Medium: 11-19
- High: 20 or more

For instance, watermelon has a high GI of 72. But because a serving of watermelon has relatively few carbohydrates, its GL is only 4, making it a low GL food.

Understanding both the GI and GL of foods can help individuals manage their blood sugar levels more effectively, particularly those with diabetes. However, these measures should be used as part of an overall balanced diet and not in isolation. It's always a good idea to consult with a healthcare professional or dietitian when making significant changes to your diet.

Chapter 2: Low Glycemic Index Diet

The Low Glycemic Index (GI) Diet is a strategic eating plan aimed at regulating blood sugar levels and promoting overall health. By prioritizing foods that have a low GI score, this diet helps to moderate the body's insulin response and maintain steady energy levels throughout the day.

Foods that have a low Glycemic Index (GI) undergo slow digestion, resulting in a steady increase in blood sugar and insulin levels. This can aid in maintaining a healthy weight and might even lower the risk of chronic illnesses. The Low GI Diet incorporates a diverse mix of whole grains, fruits, vegetables, lean meats, and beneficial fats, providing a well-rounded and sustainable path to nutritious eating. In the following section, we will explore more about the foundations and advantages of this diet.

Principles of the Low GI Diet

The Low Glycemic Index (GI) Diet is based on several key principles that guide food selection and meal planning. It's not just about choosing foods with a low GI score; it's also about balancing these choices with a nutritious, varied diet. Here are the main principles of a low GI diet:

- **Choosing Low GI Carbohydrates**: A low GI diet is fundamentally based on foods with a low glycemic index (55 or less). Such foods undergo slow digestion, triggering a steady increase in blood glucose levels. This category includes whole grains, legumes, and specific fruits and vegetables.

- **Balancing Meals with Protein and Healthy Fats**: Including a source of protein and healthy fats in meals can help further moderate blood sugar response. Proteins and fats don't have a GI score because they don't contain carbohydrates, but they can slow digestion and the absorption of sugars.
- **Eating Regular, Balanced Meals**: Regular meals prevent blood sugar dips and spikes, helping to maintain steady energy levels throughout the day. Each meal should ideally contain a balance of low GI carbohydrates, proteins, and healthy fats.
- **Portion Control**: Even foods with a low GI can lead to blood sugar spikes if eaten in large amounts. Controlling portion sizes is crucial in managing blood sugar levels and maintaining a healthy weight.
- **Including Plenty of Dietary Fiber**: High-fiber foods often have a low GI because fiber slows the digestion and absorption of carbohydrates. Foods high in dietary fiber include whole grains, fruits, vegetables, and legumes.
- **Limiting Sugary Foods and Drinks**: Sugary foods and drinks often have a high GI and can lead to rapid

blood sugar spikes. Limiting these can help maintain steady blood sugar levels.
- **Staying Hydrated**: Drinking plenty of water aids in digestion and helps maintain overall health. While water doesn't directly affect blood sugar levels, staying hydrated helps the body function optimally.

Remember, the GI of food is just one factor to consider when making dietary choices. Overall nutritional balance, individual health needs, and personal preferences should also be taken into account. Consulting with a dietitian or healthcare professional can provide personalized guidance on following a low GI diet.

Benefits of Low Glycemic Index Diet

The Low Glycemic Index (GI) Diet has been hailed for its numerous potential health benefits, which seem to significantly outweigh the few limitations associated with this diet.

- **Reduced Blood Sugar Levels**: The low GI diet is known for its ability to regulate blood sugar levels, making it particularly beneficial for those managing diabetes or prediabetes.
- **Aid in Weight Loss**: Low GI foods can promote feelings of fullness and reduce hunger, helping control caloric intake and support weight loss efforts.

- **Lower Risk of Heart Disease**: The diet encourages the consumption of whole grains, fruits, vegetables, lean proteins, and healthy fats, which contribute to heart health and may lower the risk of heart disease.
- **Sustained Energy Levels**: Foods with a low glycemic index are metabolized at a slower pace, ensuring a consistent supply of energy and preventing the sudden energy "dip" commonly associated with the intake of high-GI foods.
- **Improved Mood and Energy**: Research suggests a low GI diet could have positive effects on mood and energy, adding another potential benefit.

By incorporating low-GI foods into your diet, you can enjoy these benefits and improve your overall health. But remember, sticking to a low GI diet doesn't mean sacrificing taste or variety in your meals.

Disadvantages of a Low Glycemic Diet

Although the benefits of a low GI diet are numerous, there are some potential disadvantages to consider as well.

- **Variability in GI Values**: Different sources can list different GI values for the same food, and factors like cooking methods and ripeness can alter a food's GI.

- **Potential for Nutrient Imbalances**: If not carefully planned, focusing too strictly on GI could lead to imbalances in nutrient intake.
- **Difficulty in Identifying GI Values**: Not all foods are labeled with their GI, which can make it challenging to follow this diet consistently and accurately.

Despite these limitations, the Low GI Diet's potential health benefits appear to significantly outweigh its disadvantages. However, it's important to remember that individual health needs and goals should always be considered when deciding on any dietary plan. It is advised to consult with a healthcare professional or dietitian before starting a new diet.

Foods to Eat

The Low Glycemic Index (GI) Diet focuses on foods that have a slow impact on blood sugar levels. Here are some food options that are typically included in this diet:

- **Whole Grains**: Foods like brown rice, barley, bulgur, and oats are low GI options that can be included in meals.
- **Fruits and Vegetables**: Most fruits and non-starchy vegetables have a low GI. These include apples, oranges, peaches, berries, plums, broccoli, spinach, bell peppers, and zucchini.

- **Protein**: Lean meats, fish, eggs, legumes, and tofu have a low GI and can be a part of this diet.
- **Dairy**: Milk, cheese, yogurt, and other dairy products generally have a low GI.
- **Nuts and Seeds**: Almonds, walnuts, flaxseeds, chia seeds, and other nuts and seeds are low-GI foods that can be incorporated into meals and snacks.
- **Legumes**: Foods like black beans, lentils, chickpeas, and other legumes are low GI options.

It's important to remember that the Low GI Diet is not just about choosing low GI foods, but also about balancing these with moderate and high GI foods to maintain a healthy and varied diet. For a more personalized plan, it's recommended to consult with a dietitian or healthcare professional.

Foods to Avoid

When following a Low Glycemic Index (GI) Diet, certain foods that have a high GI should be limited or avoided. These include:

- **Refined Grains**: White bread, white rice, and other refined grains can have a high GI and should be limited.
- **Sugary Drinks**: Beverages like soda, sweetened iced tea, and fruit drinks often have a high GI due to the added sugars.

- **Sweet Treats and Desserts**: Pastries, cakes, cookies, candy, and other sweet treats typically have a high GI and should be eaten sparingly.
- **Certain Fruits and Vegetables**: While most fruits and vegetables have a low GI, some, like watermelon, pineapple, and potatoes, can have a high GI.
- **Processed Foods**: Many processed foods, such as chips, crackers, and instant meals, can have a high GI.
- **Certain Breakfast Cereals**: Some breakfast cereals, especially those that are highly processed or contain added sugars, can have a high GI.

It's important to note that having a balanced diet is key. This means that while these high-GI foods should be limited, they don't necessarily need to be completely eliminated. It's also recommended to consult with a healthcare professional or a dietitian for personalized dietary advice.

Now that you know more about Low Glycemic Index and how it works, allow me to walk you through the step-by-step guide on starting your own LGI diet.

I have designed a 3-week guide that you can use to start the Low Glycemic Index Diet and make it your new eating habit.

Chapter 3: Week 1: Getting Started

The first week is the preparation week. Before we start, let's do some pre-LGI diet checks and preparation. You can incorporate the low glycemic diet program with your current diet regimen. If your doctor or nutritionist prescribed a diet regimen for you, there is no need to change it.

Keep in mind that low glycemic diet is not about dieting. It is making smart food choices that will help lower your blood sugar levels. Your meal should still be within the context of your prescribed diet. It is best to consult your physician or nutritionist before embarking on this diet.

List down your current diet / current food list

Week 1 of your journey towards a healthier lifestyle involves analyzing your current diet and comparing it to the principles of a Low Glycemic Index (GI) Diet. This process will help you understand where you can make beneficial changes.

To start, jot down every item in your current diet.

Don't leave anything out – from your morning coffee or tea to that midnight snack. It's crucial to be honest with yourself here. You need to know exactly what you're consuming to make effective changes.

Next, delve deeper into your foods by listing out their individual ingredients.

If you're eating pre-packaged or processed foods, this might mean reading labels. If you're cooking at home, list out each component of your meals.

Now, it's time to cross-reference these ingredients with their glycemic index values.

The glycemic index is a tool that gauges the speed at which food escalates blood glucose levels. Foods that have a low GI score (ranging from 0-55) undergo slower digestion, leading to a steady elevation in blood sugar levels. You can look up the GI scores of most foods on the internet.

Compare each ingredient's GI value against your list. Mark ingredients with a GI higher than 55. These are the foods to limit or replace with lower GI alternatives.

Remember, not all food groups have a GI value. Foods with little to no carbs like meat, seafood, fats, oils, nuts, and certain herbs/spices won't have a GI value. You can freely include these in your low GI diet.

For example, protein sources like beef, pork, chicken, lamb, eggs, and seafood like salmon, tuna, trout, sardines, and prawns. Healthy fats and oils like olive oil, butter, margarine, and rice bran oil are also fine. Nuts including cashews, almonds, walnuts, pistachios, and macadamia nuts, along with herbs and spices like salt, pepper, basil, dill, and garlic, can be incorporated into meals.

If you can't find the GI value for certain foods, reliable sources like Health Harvard Glycemic Index Listing and Glycemic Index Food Listing can help.

This exercise isn't just about eliminating high GI foods but understanding how foods affect blood sugar levels and health. Once you have this info, you can make informed decisions and gradually shift to a low GI diet. Remember, it's about progress, not perfection. Small, consistent changes can lead to significant long-term benefits.

Find alternative food for high-value numbers

After comparing your food list with glycemic index values, you may notice some foods outside the low GI range. But don't panic! Many high-GI foods can be replaced with delicious and healthier alternatives, allowing you to maintain a varied diet.

Not all carbohydrates are equal. Some are high in sugar, resulting in a high GI value, while others have lower sugar content and a correspondingly lower GI value. This is where substitutions come into play.

Take ice cream, for example. Although it falls into the low GI category with a value of 51, it's high in fat and sugar, making it less ideal for overall health. Fruit yogurt, with a lower GI value of 41, is a better option.

Substituting ice cream with fruit yogurt reduces the GI value and offers additional health benefits. Fruit yogurt has less fat and sugar, and it's a good source of gut-friendly probiotics. The fruit adds fiber, further lowering the effective GI and providing essential nutrients.

The goal is to make smarter choices that support your health without depriving yourself. It's about finding balance and enjoying food with a healthier twist.

Remember to consult with a healthcare professional or dietitian for personalized dietary advice. They can guide you on suitable low GI substitutions based on your needs and preferences.

Finalizing your list

It's time to finalize your food list. When doing so, remember that a low glycemic diet isn't just about GI values. It's equally important to choose foods you enjoy eating. After all, sticking to a diet is easier when you love the food.

For example, if apples (GI=36) aren't your thing, don't force yourself to eat them just because of their low GI value.

Instead, opt for a fruit you genuinely enjoy, like an orange (GI=43). It might have a slightly higher GI value, but what matters is that you're eating healthy and enjoying it.

Consider your dietary restrictions and personal preferences too. If you're lactose intolerant or don't like milk, there are plenty of alternatives available. Soy milk, for example, can be a great substitute and it's low GI too.

Remember, unless you're following a prescribed diet, a low glycemic diet doesn't need to be overly strict. Choose foods that won't cause a rapid increase in your blood sugar levels and are within an acceptable glycemic load.

It's not just about the numbers. Find a balance between steady blood sugar levels, meeting nutritional needs, and enjoying what you eat. This approach helps build a sustainable eating habit rather than a temporary diet.

As always, consult with a healthcare professional or dietitian for personalized advice. They can help create a balanced, low-GI diet plan that suits your tastes, meets your nutritional needs, and aligns with any dietary restrictions you may have. With their guidance and your new knowledge of the glycemic index, you're well-equipped to make informed decisions about your diet.

Chapter 4: Week 2: Creating Your Meal Plan

A meal plan serves as a guide, outlining the food you can consume during each meal. A typical meal includes breakfast, a morning snack, lunch, an afternoon snack, dinner, and an optional nighttime snack.

You have the flexibility to create a 7-day, 14-day, or even a 30-day meal plan, depending on your preference. For this exercise, we'll focus on a 5-day plan, designed to be easily adjustable. It's important to introduce dietary changes gradually, allowing your body to adapt to new eating habits. Unlike fad diets that impose drastic adjustments, this approach promotes sustainable progress, reducing the temptation to cheat or give up.

Creating your recipes

You'll find many low-glycemic recipes that you can find online. You can also use non-low glycemic recipes and substitute the ingredients with low glycemic alternatives.

Checking the calories and macronutrient count

When crafting your meal plan, it's not just about focusing on low glycemic index foods. It's crucial to also consider calorie count and macronutrient distribution. According to the USDA

Dietary Guidelines, the standard daily caloric intake for maintaining weight is around 2,000 calories, while a 1,500-calorie daily intake can lead to a weight loss of approximately one pound per week. However, remember that these are general guidelines and actual needs may vary based on factors such as age, height, current weight, activity levels, metabolic health, and more.

Nowadays, you'll find many recipes online that already include both calorie count and macronutrient breakdown. This makes it easier for you to align your meals with your dietary goals. By checking the GI for each ingredient in the recipe, you can calculate the total Glycemic Load (GL) based on the calorie count per serving.

Remember the GL equation we discussed in Chapter 1? You'll use this to determine the GL of each meal you prepare. While the glycemic index is the primary factor in a low glycemic diet, monitoring the glycemic load of your food intake is also important.

The glycemic load gives you a more accurate picture of how a specific food or meal will impact your blood sugar levels, taking into account not just the type of carbohydrate, but also the quantity. This way, you can ensure you're not only eating low-GI foods but also controlling the overall impact on your blood sugar levels.

Remember, balance is key. A healthy, sustainable meal plan should include a variety of foods that you enjoy, meet your caloric and nutritional needs, and help maintain stable blood sugar levels. Always consult with a healthcare professional or dietitian to ensure your meal plan is tailored to your individual needs and goals.

Make your shopping list

Once you have your recipes, it's time to go grocery shopping. The good news is, you don't have to make drastic changes to your shopping routine. The key difference now is that you'll need to focus on selecting food groups and ingredients with low glycemic readings. Gone are the days of grabbing whatever you want from the shelves.

Before heading to the grocery store, make a list of all the ingredients needed for your recipes. Chances are, some ingredients will overlap across different recipes. By buying these items in bulk, you can save both money and time.

It's advisable to do your shopping before finalizing your meal plan. This way, you can ensure that all the necessary ingredients are available. It's much easier to adjust your meal plans based on what's in stock, rather than scrambling to find specific ingredients, which can be both expensive and time-consuming.

During your grocery trip, you may encounter certain ingredients that are only available in canned or processed forms. Determining the glycemic value of such products can be challenging.

However, here are a few tips to consider:

- **Check the** carbohydrate-to-protein **and Fat Ratio:** If the ratio of carbohydrates is relatively low compared to protein and fats, then the food is likely to have a low glycemic index.
- **Consider Total Carbohydrates:** Keep in mind that total carbohydrates listed on food labels typically include both starch and sugars. Fiber is often removed during processing.
- **Look for High Fiber Content:** Foods with high fiber content, especially soluble fiber, usually have a low glycemic index value.
- **Search for the GI Symbol:** Look out for the Glycemic Index symbol on food packaging. This symbol guarantees that the food has a low glycemic index.

By following these guidelines, you can make informed choices while grocery shopping and maintain a meal plan that aligns with your dietary needs.

Creating Your Meal Plan

So now, it's time to create your meal plan. As mentioned, for this exercise we will start with a 5-day meal plan consisting of breakfast, lunch, dinner and two snacks. If you have a prescribed meal plan, stick with it. Just substitute the food items or ingredients with a low glycemic value.

Day 1

Breakfast

- 1 bowl of Quinoa and black beans
- 2 slices of low-sodium bacon,
- ½ cup Orange Juice

AM Snack

- 1 mozzarella cheese stick
- 8 oz. water

Lunch

- 1 halve-side Crab Stuff Avocado
- 2 slices toast wheat bread

PM Snack

- 1 small peach
- 8 oz. water

Dinner

- 1 cup fruit salad (kiwi, apple, orange, grapefruit)
- 1 serving Lemon Chicken Salad
- 1 slice of barley bread
- 8 oz. water

Day 2

Breakfast

- ½ cup Quinoa Porridge with ½ cup raspberries,
- 2 slices turkey bacon,
- 8 oz. coffee with almond milk

AM Snack

- 6 almond flour crackers with 1 tbsp.
- peanut butter
- 8 oz. water

Lunch

- Beef Stew
- 2 slices rye bread

PM Snack

- 1 pear
- 8 oz. water

Dinner

- Tomato & Basil Soup
- 1 cup steamed cauliflower
- 1 almond muffin
- 8 oz. water

Day 3

Breakfast

- 1 bowl apple muesli
- 2 poached eggs
- 8 oz. unsweetened iced tea

AM Snack

- 6 oz. yogurt with ½ cup strawberries
- 8 oz. water

Lunch

- Grilled tenderloin
- ½ cup mixed lettuce onion
- tomato with vinaigrette

PM Snack

- 1 small apple, 8 oz. water

Dinner

- 1 bowl mixed green salad with apple cider

- 1 slice grilled salmon with lemon
- 8 oz. protein shake
- 8 oz. water

Day 4

Breakfast

- 1 piece buckwheat pancake with blueberries
- 2 boiled eggs
- ½ large grapefruit
- 8 oz. coffee with skim milk and stevia

AM Snack

- 2 slices cinnamon and almond loaf
- 8 oz. water

Lunch

- Braised balsamic chicken
- 2 slices wheat bread

PM Snack

- ½ cup strawberries
- 8 oz. water

Dinner

- 1 serving beef and mushroom pie,

- 1 cup steamed broccoli,
- 1 tub Greek yogurt
- 8 oz. water

Day 5

Breakfast

- 50 grams salmon with 2 scrambled eggs
- ½ medium banana
- 8 oz. coffee with skim milk and stevia

AM Snack

- 8 oz. strawberry and yogurt crunch
- 8 oz. water

Lunch

- 1 lean roast beef sandwich in barley bread
- 1 cup steamed broccoli

PM Snack

- 1 orange
- 8 oz. water

Dinner

- 1 grilled lamb
- ½ cup basmati rice

- 1 cup steamed green beans,
- 4 whole grain crackers with low-fat cream cheese
- 8 oz. water

Remember to drink plenty of water throughout the day to stay well-hydrated!

Chapter 5: Sample Recipes

Crab Stuffed Avocados

Ingredients:

- 2 ripe avocados
- 1 cup of lump crabmeat
- 1/4 cup of diced red onion
- 1/4 cup of diced red bell pepper
- 1/4 cup of chopped fresh cilantro
- 1 lime, juiced
- Salt and pepper to taste
- 1 tablespoon of olive oil

Instructions:

1. Slice the avocados in half lengthwise and remove the pits. Scoop out a bit of the flesh in the center to make room for the crab stuffing. Set aside.
2. In a bowl, combine the crabmeat, red onion, red bell pepper, and cilantro. Mix well.
3. Pour the lime juice over the crab mixture, then drizzle with olive oil. Season with salt and pepper to taste. Stir until all the ingredients are well combined.
4. Spoon an equal amount of the crab mixture into each avocado half.
5. Serve immediately and enjoy!

Beef Stew

Ingredients:

- 1.5 lbs of lean beef stew meat, cut into 1-inch cubes
- Salt and pepper to taste
- 2 tablespoons of olive oil
- 1 large onion, chopped
- 3 cloves of garlic, minced
- 4 cups of low-sodium beef broth
- 2 carrots, peeled and sliced into 1-inch pieces
- 2 parsnips, peeled and cut into 1-inch cubes (parsnips have a lower glycemic index than potatoes)
- 1 bay leaf
- 1 teaspoon of dried thyme
- 1 cup of frozen green peas (green peas have a lower glycemic index than other types of peas)
- 1 cup of diced tomatoes

Instructions:

1. Season the beef with salt and pepper.
2. Heat the olive oil in a large pot over medium-high heat. Add the beef and brown on all sides. Remove the beef from the pot and set aside.
3. In the same pot, add the onion and cook until softened. Add the garlic and cook for another minute.
4. Return the beef to the pot, then add the beef broth, carrots, parsnips, bay leaf, and thyme. Stir well.

5. Bring the mixture to a boil, then reduce the heat to low, cover, and simmer for about 2 hours, or until the beef is tender.
6. Add the frozen green peas and diced tomatoes and cook for another 10 minutes.
7. Taste and adjust the seasoning with more salt and pepper if needed.
8. Serve hot.

Lemon Chicken Salad

Ingredients:

- 2 boneless, skinless chicken breasts
- Salt and pepper to taste
- 1 tablespoon of olive oil
- Juice and zest of 1 lemon
- 1 clove of garlic, minced
- 1 teaspoon of Dijon mustard
- 1/4 cup of extra-virgin olive oil
- 6 cups of mixed salad greens
- 1 cucumber, sliced
- 1 bell pepper, sliced
- 1/4 cup of almonds, toasted

Instructions:

1. Season the chicken breasts with salt and pepper.

2. Heat the olive oil in a skillet over medium heat. Add the chicken and cook for 6-7 minutes on each side, or until cooked through. Remove from the heat and let it cool.
3. While the chicken is cooling, make the dressing. In a small bowl, combine the lemon juice, lemon zest, garlic, and Dijon mustard. Gradually whisk in the extra-virgin olive oil until the dressing is emulsified. Season with salt and pepper to taste.
4. Slice the cooled chicken into thin strips.
5. In a large bowl, combine the salad greens, cucumber, bell pepper, and chicken. Drizzle with the dressing and toss to coat.
6. Sprinkle the toasted almonds on top.
7. Serve immediately.

Grilled Tenderloin

Ingredients:

- 1 pork or beef tenderloin (about 1 to 1.5 lbs)
- Salt and pepper to taste
- 2 tablespoons of olive oil
- 2 cloves of garlic, minced
- 1 teaspoon of dried rosemary
- 1 teaspoon of dried thyme

For the side dish:

- 2 zucchinis, sliced
- 1 bell pepper, cut into strips
- 1 tablespoon of olive oil
- Salt and pepper to taste

Instructions:

1. Set your grill to preheat at a medium-high temperature.
2. Season the tenderloin with salt and pepper. In a small bowl, mix together the olive oil, garlic, rosemary, and thyme. Rub this mixture all over the tenderloin.
1. Place the tenderloin on the grill and cook for about 20-25 minutes, turning occasionally, until the internal temperature reaches 145°F for pork or 160°F for beef.
2. While the tenderloin is grilling, toss the zucchini and bell pepper with the olive oil, salt, and pepper. Grill these alongside the tenderloin for about 10 minutes, or until they are tender and slightly charred.
3. Remove the tenderloin from the grill and let it rest for a few minutes before slicing.
4. Serve the sliced tenderloin with the grilled vegetables on the side.

Quinoa and Black Beans

Ingredients:

- 1 cup of quinoa
- 2 cups of water

- 1 tablespoon olive oil
- 1 onion, diced
- 3 cloves garlic, minced
- 1 can (15 oz) black beans, drained and rinsed
- 1 teaspoon cumin
- 1/2 teaspoon chili powder
- Salt and pepper to taste
- Juice of 1 lime
- 1/4 cup of fresh chopped cilantro

Instructions:

1. Rinse the quinoa under cold water until the water runs clear. This helps remove any bitterness.
2. In a saucepan, bring the 2 cups of water to a boil. Add the quinoa, reduce heat to low, cover, and let it simmer for about 15 minutes, or until the quinoa is tender and the water has been absorbed. Remove from heat and let it sit covered for 5 minutes.
3. While the quinoa is cooking, heat the olive oil in a skillet over medium heat. Add the onion and sauté until it's soft and translucent. Add the garlic and cook for another minute.
4. Stir in the black beans, cumin, chili powder, and salt and pepper. Cook for a few minutes until everything is well combined and heated through.
5. Fluff the cooked quinoa with a fork, then add it to the skillet. Stir to combine.

6. Drizzle the lime juice over the quinoa and bean mixture, then sprinkle with the chopped cilantro.
7. Serve warm.

Braised Balsamic Chicken

Ingredients:

- 6 skinless, boneless chicken breasts
- Salt and pepper to taste
- 2 teaspoons garlic powder
- 1 tablespoon olive oil
- 1 onion, thinly sliced
- 3 cloves of garlic, minced
- 1 can (14.5 oz) diced tomatoes
- 1/2 cup balsamic vinegar
- 1 teaspoon dried basil
- 1 teaspoon dried oregano
- 1 teaspoon dried rosemary
- 1/2 teaspoon dried thyme

Instructions:

1. Season both sides of the chicken breasts with salt, pepper, and garlic powder.
2. Heat the olive oil in a skillet over medium heat. Add the chicken and cook until it's browned on both sides. Remove the chicken from the skillet and set it aside.

3. In the same skillet, add the onion and garlic. Cook until the onion is translucent.
4. Add the diced tomatoes, balsamic vinegar, basil, oregano, rosemary, and thyme to the skillet. Stir well to combine.
5. Return the chicken to the skillet, making sure to coat it with the sauce.
6. Reduce the heat to low, cover the skillet, and let it simmer for about 20-25 minutes, or until the chicken is cooked through.
7. Serve the chicken hot, spooning the sauce over the top

Tomato and Basil Soup

Ingredients:

- 1 tablespoon olive oil
- 1 onion, diced
- 2 garlic cloves, minced
- 1 can (28 ounces) of no-sugar-added diced tomatoes
- 2 cups of low-sodium vegetable broth
- Salt and pepper to taste
- 1/4 cup fresh basil leaves, chopped
- 1/2 cup of heavy cream

Instructions:

1. Heat the olive oil in a large pot over medium heat. Add the onion and cook until it's soft and translucent.

2. Add the garlic and cook for another minute, until it's fragrant.
3. Stir in the diced tomatoes, vegetable broth, salt, and pepper. Bring the mixture to a boil.
4. Reduce the heat to low and let it simmer for about 15 minutes, or until the flavors have melded together.
5. Stir in the chopped basil leaves.
6. Use an immersion blender to puree the soup until it's smooth. If you don't have an immersion blender, you can also carefully transfer the soup to a regular blender to puree it.
7. Stir in the heavy cream and heat through.
8. Serve hot, garnishing with additional fresh basil if desired.

Lean Roast Beef Sandwich on Barley Bread

Ingredients:

- 2 slices of barley bread
- 3 ounces of lean roast beef, thinly sliced
- 1 slice of low-fat cheese (optional)
- Lettuce leaves
- 2-3 slices of tomato
- 1/4 of an avocado, sliced
- 1 tablespoon of low-fat mayonnaise or mustard
- Salt and pepper to taste

Instructions:

1. Lay out the two slices of barley bread.
2. Spread one side of each slice with the low-fat mayonnaise or mustard.
3. On one slice of bread, arrange the lettuce leaves, tomato slices, and avocado slices.
4. Layer the thinly sliced roast beef over the vegetables. If using, place the slice of low-fat cheese on top of the roast beef.
5. Sprinkle with a pinch of salt and pepper to taste.
6. Top with the second slice of bread.
7. Cut the sandwich in half if desired, and serve.

Beef and Mushroom Pie

Ingredients:

For the filling:

- 500g lean beef, cut into chunks
- 2 tablespoons olive oil
- 1 large onion, chopped
- 2 cloves garlic, minced
- 200g mushrooms, sliced
- 2 tablespoons tomato paste
- 1 cup beef broth, low-sodium
- Salt and pepper to taste
- 1 teaspoon dried thyme

- 1 teaspoon dried rosemary

For the crust:

- 1 cup almond flour
- 1/4 cup coconut flour
- 1/2 teaspoon salt
- 1/2 cup butter, chilled and diced
- 1 egg

Instructions:

1. Heat the olive oil in a large pan over medium heat. Add the beef and cook until browned. Remove and set aside.
2. In the same pan, add the onion and garlic. Cook until translucent.
3. Add the mushrooms and cook until they have released their juices.
4. Stir in the tomato paste, beef broth, salt, pepper, thyme, and rosemary. Bring to a boil.
5. Return the beef to the pan, reduce the heat to low, cover, and simmer for about 1 hour or until the beef is tender.
6. While the filling is cooking, prepare the crust. In a large bowl, mix together the almond flour, coconut flour, and salt.

7. Add the chilled, diced butter to the flour mixture. Use your fingers to rub the butter into the flour until the mixture resembles coarse breadcrumbs.
8. Stir in the egg until a dough forms.
9. Preheat your oven to 180°C (350°F).
10. Once the filling is done, pour it into a pie dish.
11. Roll out the dough between two pieces of parchment paper to the size of your pie dish.
12. Carefully place the dough over the filling, pressing it down at the edges to seal.
13. Bake for 20-25 minutes, or until the crust is golden.
14. Allow to cool for a few minutes before serving.

Grilled Lamb

Ingredients:

- 4 lamb chops
- 2 tablespoons olive oil
- 2 cloves of garlic, minced
- 1 teaspoon dried rosemary
- Salt and pepper to taste
- Lemon wedges, for serving

Instructions:

1. Rinse the lamb chops under cold water and pat dry with paper towels.

2. In a small bowl, combine the olive oil, minced garlic, dried rosemary, salt, and pepper.
3. Rub this mixture all over the lamb chops, ensuring they're well-coated.
4. Allow the lamb chops to marinate for at least 30 minutes. If you have time, letting them marinate for a few hours in the refrigerator can enhance the flavor.
5. Set your grill to preheat at a medium-high temperature.
6. Place the lamb chops on the grill. Cook for about 3-4 minutes on each side for medium-rare, or until they reach your desired level of doneness.
7. Remove the lamb chops from the grill and let them rest for a few minutes before serving.
8. Serve the grilled lamb with fresh lemon wedges.

Buckwheat Pancakes with Blueberries

Ingredients:

- 1 cup buckwheat flour
- 1 tablespoon baking powder
- 1/2 teaspoon salt
- 1 tablespoon Stevia (or other non-nutritive sweetener)
- 1 cup almond milk (unsweetened)
- 1 large egg
- 2 tablespoons coconut oil (melted and cooled)
- 1/2 teaspoon pure vanilla extract
- 1 cup fresh blueberries

Instructions:

1. In a large bowl, combine the buckwheat flour, baking powder, salt, and Stevia.
2. In another bowl, whisk together the almond milk, egg, melted coconut oil, and vanilla extract.
3. Pour the wet ingredients into the dry ingredients and stir until just combined.
4. Gently fold in the fresh blueberries.
5. Heat a non-stick skillet or griddle over medium heat.
6. Pour 1/4 cup of batter for each pancake onto the skillet.
7. Cook until bubbles form on the surface of the pancake and the edges look set, about 2-3 minutes.
8. Flip the pancake and cook for another 2-3 minutes or until golden brown and cooked through.
9. Repeat with the remaining batter.
10. Serve the pancakes warm. Add a dollop of Greek yogurt or a drizzle of sugar-free syrup if desired.

Almond Butter Banana Smoothie

Ingredients:

- 1 ripe banana
- 2 tablespoons almond butter
- 1 cup unsweetened almond milk
- A handful of ice cubes

Instructions:

1. Peel the banana and break it into chunks.
2. Put the banana pieces in a blender.
3. Add the almond butter to the blender.
4. Pour in the unsweetened almond milk.
5. Add a handful of ice cubes.
6. Blend all the ingredients together until smooth and creamy. This should take about 1-2 minutes depending on your blender.
7. Pour the smoothie into a glass and enjoy immediately.

Grilled Eggplant and Zucchini Salad

Ingredients:

- 1 large eggplant
- 2 medium zucchinis
- 2 tablespoons olive oil
- Sea salt and ground black pepper to taste
- Juice of 1 lemon
- A handful of fresh basil leaves

Instructions:

1. Set your grill to preheat at a medium-high temperature.
2. Slice the eggplant and zucchinis lengthwise into 1/4-inch thick slices. Brush both sides of the vegetable

slices with olive oil and season with sea salt and black pepper.
3. Place the eggplant and zucchini slices on the grill. Grill for about 3-4 minutes per side, or until they have nice grill marks and are tender and slightly charred.
4. Once the vegetables are grilled, transfer them to a serving platter. Drizzle the grilled vegetables with lemon juice.
5. Tear the basil leaves and scatter them over the grilled vegetables.
6. The salad can be served warm, or you can let it cool to room temperature.

Sweet Potato and Black Bean Tacos

Ingredients:

- 2 medium sweet potatoes, peeled and cubed
- 1 can (15 oz) black beans, drained and rinsed
- 1 medium onion, finely chopped
- 2 cloves garlic, minced
- 1 teaspoon ground cumin
- Salt and pepper to taste
- 8 small corn tortillas
- Fresh cilantro leaves for garnish
- 1 lime, cut into wedges

Instructions:

1. Heat a bit of olive oil in a large skillet over medium heat. Add the onion and garlic, sautéing until they start to soften.
2. Add the cubed sweet potatoes to the skillet, stirring to mix them with the onions and garlic. Cover the skillet and let it cook for about 10 minutes, or until the sweet potatoes are tender. You may want to stir occasionally to prevent them from sticking to the skillet.
3. Once the sweet potatoes are tender, stir in the black beans, cumin, salt, and pepper. Cook for another 5 minutes until everything is heated through.
4. While the sweet potato and black bean mixture is cooking, warm up your corn tortillas. You can do this in a dry skillet over medium heat, flipping them over after about 30 seconds on each side.
5. To serve, spoon the sweet potato and black bean mixture onto the warm corn tortillas. Garnish with fresh cilantro leaves and squeeze a wedge of lime over the top for added flavor.

Chickpea and Kale Curry

Ingredients:

- 1 can (15 oz) chickpeas, drained and rinsed
- 2 cups chopped kale
- 1 medium onion, finely chopped
- 2 cloves garlic, minced

- 1 tablespoon curry powder
- 1 can (13.5 oz) coconut milk
- Salt to taste
- 1 tablespoon olive oil

Instructions:

1. Heat the olive oil in a large pot over medium heat. Add the onion and garlic, and sauté until they start to soften.
2. Stir in the curry powder, mixing it with the onions and garlic. Cook for a minute until the curry powder is fragrant.
3. Add the drained and rinsed chickpeas to the pot. Stir everything together so that the chickpeas are coated in the curry powder.
4. Pour in the coconut milk, stirring to combine. Bring the mixture to a simmer.
5. Once simmering, add the chopped kale to the pot. Stir it into the curry, then cover the pot. Let the curry simmer for about 10 minutes, or until the kale is wilted and tender.
6. Taste the curry and add salt as needed.
7. Serve your Chickpea and Kale Curry hot, over a bed of cooked brown rice or quinoa if desired.

Chapter 6: Week 3: Evaluation and Adjustments

Welcome to Week 3 of your Low Glycemic Index Diet journey. It's time to put your well-thought-out meal plan into action, monitor your progress, and make needed adjustments. Here's a step-by-step guide for you.

Keeping a Record

Keeping a detailed record is crucial for managing your Low Glycemic Index Diet. It tracks your progress, helps you understand the impact of your meal plan on your health, and allows you to make necessary adjustments for optimal results.

To start your third week, set up a dedicated record book. It doesn't have to be fancy - a simple notebook will do. Use it as a central location to jot down and review important details about your journey.

On the first page, write your current weight and fasting blood sugar level as baseline measurements. Take these measurements in the morning, before eating or drinking anything, for accuracy.

From the second day onwards, start each day with a fasting blood sugar test before breakfast. Repeat the test after lunch and dinner. This helps you understand how your meals affect your blood sugar levels.

Record all these readings in your book. Also note what you eat, any physical activity, and your overall feelings. This additional information helps you identify patterns, understand the effects of different foods, and make informed decisions about your diet.

Remember, the goal is to understand your body's response, not achieve perfection. Learn from experiences and use them to improve your diet and health.

Implementing Your Meal Plan

As you embark on this exciting journey towards improved health, the implementation of your meal plan is an essential step. This isn't just about following a diet - it's about making a lifestyle change that could have a significant impact on your overall well-being.

Staying vigilant is key during this time. This doesn't mean you should be overly rigid or critical, but rather, you should be mindful and attentive to your body's signals. Are you feeling satisfied after meals, or do you find yourself still hungry? Do certain foods make you feel more energized than others? Noticing these subtle cues can help you fine-tune your meal plan to better suit your needs and preferences.

It's also important to remember that cravings are a normal part of the process, especially during the initial adjustment period. You're introducing new foods to your diet and reducing or eliminating others, and your body may naturally react to these changes. Cravings don't mean you're failing or that the diet isn't working. Instead, see them as an opportunity to explore new, low-glycemic alternatives to the foods you're missing.

For example, if you're craving something sweet, consider having a piece of fruit or a small portion of dark chocolate instead of reaching for a sugary dessert. If you're missing pasta, try spaghetti squash or spiralized zucchini as a low-glycemic alternative.

As you implement your meal plan, remember to be patient with yourself. It takes time for your body to adjust to a new way of eating, and there might be some trial and error involved. What matters is that you're making a conscious effort to improve your health, and every step you take in the right direction counts.

By staying vigilant, paying attention to your body, and being flexible in your approach, you'll be well on your way to successfully implementing your Low Glycemic Index Diet.

Making Necessary Adjustments

Making necessary adjustments to your diet is a critical aspect of managing your blood sugar levels, especially when following a Low Glycemic Index (GI) Diet. This diet involves consuming foods that have a lesser impact on blood sugar levels, but that doesn't mean you can set it and forget it. You'll need to be proactive in monitoring your blood sugar levels to ensure they're staying within the ideal range.

For those unfamiliar with the process, monitoring blood sugar levels involves using a blood glucose meter, which requires a small blood sample. The frequency of checks varies depending on individual health status and doctor's recommendations. However, it's generally beneficial to check these levels before meals and two hours after eating.

If you find that your blood sugar levels are dropping too quickly, it might indicate that your body needs more carbohydrates than you're currently providing. On the other hand, if your blood sugar levels aren't decreasing at all or are increasing, it could mean that you're consuming too many carbs or the ones with a high glycemic index. In either case, you'll need to adjust your meal plan accordingly.

Keep in mind that the primary objective of adhering to a Low GI Diet is to sustain consistent and healthy blood glucose levels. It's not about significantly cutting down your carbohydrate consumption, but instead, it's about selecting the appropriate types of carbs - those that undergo slow digestion and absorption, leading to a gradual and minor increase in blood sugar levels.

For non-diabetics, blood sugar levels should ideally range between 60-90 mg/dl before meals. Two hours after eating, these levels should be less than 140 mg/dl. These numbers serve as a good benchmark for those looking to maintain a healthy lifestyle and prevent future health issues related to blood sugar control.

For diabetics, the ranges slightly differ. The ideal range before meals is 70-130 mg/dl, and less than 180 mg/dl two hours post-meal. These targets might vary based on factors like age, pregnancy, and overall health, so it's always best to consult with a healthcare professional for personalized advice.

Adjusting your diet according to your monitored blood sugar levels is crucial in reaping the benefits of a Low GI Diet. It's a continuous process of learning and fine-tuning what works best for your body. So, keep monitoring, keep adjusting, and keep striving for better health.

Evaluating Your Progress

Five days into the Low Glycemic Diet, it's time to take a moment and evaluate your progress. Step on the scale and observe any changes. Remember, the primary focus of this diet isn't about shedding pounds; it's about embracing a healthier lifestyle. Any weight loss you experience is merely an added benefit.

Take some time to introspect. Reflect on how the past few days have been for you. Have you noticed any changes in your energy levels or mood since you began the diet? Are there certain foods you're enjoying more than others? Are there any challenges you're facing in sticking to the diet? These are all important aspects to consider when evaluating your progress.

Don't hesitate to experiment with the parameters of the diet. The beauty of the Low Glycemic Diet is its flexibility. While it's crucial to adhere to the basic principles, such as prioritizing low-glycemic foods, there's a wealth of variety available to you. Try new fruits and vegetables, experiment with different whole grains, or explore recipes that incorporate more legumes.

Remember, the aim isn't just to follow the diet rigidly but to incorporate it into your lifestyle in a way that's enjoyable and sustainable for you. So, if you find that certain foods or meals aren't working for you, don't be afraid to switch them up.

Lastly, keep in mind that change takes time. You might not see immediate results, but that doesn't mean the diet isn't working. Consistency is key here, so stick with it and remember to be patient with yourself. This isn't just a diet—it's a journey towards a healthier you.

Importance of Record Keeping

When embarking on your journey with new dietary habits, such as the Low Glycemic Index Diet, the importance of keeping a record cannot be overstated. It serves as a tangible and reliable tool that helps you navigate this lifestyle change more effectively.

Firstly, record-keeping allows you to track your progress in a measurable way. By noting down your weight, blood sugar levels, and even subjective observations about how you feel, you can map out your journey and see how far you've come. This can be incredibly motivating and can help you stay committed to your diet plan.

Secondly, maintaining a record helps you identify what's working for you and what isn't. Every individual is unique, and what works well for one person may not work as well for another. By keeping a record of your meals, their glycemic index, and your subsequent blood sugar readings, you can identify patterns and understand which foods your body reacts well to.

Finally, this record becomes the basis for informed decision-making. If you notice that certain meals spike your blood sugar levels, you can decide to replace or reduce these in your meal plan. Similarly, if some foods keep you satiated for longer and don't cause significant blood sugar fluctuations, you'd know to include them more frequently.

Planning Ahead

As you approach the end of week 3, it's time to look ahead and start preparing your meal plan for the upcoming period. This is a crucial step in maintaining consistency and ensuring the success of your new dietary lifestyle.

Whether you choose to plan your meals on a weekly or bi-weekly basis is entirely dependent on what works best for you. However, it's worth noting that a longer-term plan—such as planning for two weeks at a time—can often prove to be more cost-effective. By planning and shopping in larger quantities, you can take advantage of bulk discounts and reduce the number of trips you make to the grocery store.

Moreover, having a longer-term plan in place can help you adhere to your new diet more effectively. With a clear plan, you'll know exactly what you're eating each day, eliminating the daily stress of deciding what to cook. It also reduces the temptation to deviate from your diet, as you've already dedicated time and resources to preparing your meals.

Remember, the goal of planning ahead isn't just about being organized—it's about setting yourself up for success on your journey towards a healthier lifestyle. With a well-planned menu, you're one step closer to achieving your health and wellness goals.

Chapter 7: The Last Step: Make it a Habit

The final and perhaps most challenging phase in our journey is transforming the Low Glycemic Diet into a sustainable lifestyle. It's not just about planning, testing, and evaluating; it's about maintaining this new way of eating consistently.

Practical Tips for Sustaining a Low Glycemic Diet

Transforming the Low Glycemic Diet into a habit may seem daunting, but it's actually quite manageable. The beauty of this diet is that it still allows you to enjoy your favorite foods, albeit with some limitations. Here are some practical strategies to help you sustain a Low Glycemic Diet:

- **Prioritize non-starchy vegetables and fruits:** Opt for leafy greens, legumes, and low-glycemic fruits like apples, oranges, peaches, and berries.
- **Choose whole grains:** Instead of white bread, go for barley, whole wheat, or sourdough. These options have a lower glycemic index.
- **Rethink breakfast:** Swap sugary cereals for oatmeal, porridge, or natural muesli. If you must have cereal, choose brands that are specifically marked as low GI.
- **Select healthy fats:** Incorporate olive oil, nuts (like walnuts, almonds, pecans), and avocados into your diet, but do so in moderation.

- **Limit sugary treats:** Try to reduce your intake of desserts like ice cream and sweetened beverages like fruit juices.
- **Consume protein-rich foods:** Include moderate amounts of meat, fish, seafood, and poultry in your meals.
- **Use acid to your advantage:** Foods with high acid content, such as sourdough, oranges, and vinaigrette, can slow down the conversion of carbohydrates into sugar, thus lowering their glycemic count.
- **Be mindful of cooking methods:** Generally, raw foods have a lower glycemic index than cooked ones.

Dining Out

Dining out, while enjoyable and social, can often pose challenges for those following a specific diet, like the Low Glycemic Diet. The lack of control over meal preparation and ingredients can make it feel daunting. However, with an increasing number of restaurants offering health-conscious options, it's becoming easier to dine out without compromising on your dietary needs.

One of the key things to remember when dining out is that you can still make informed choices. For instance, you could opt for sit-down restaurants instead of fast food chains. Fast food tends to be high in carbohydrates and unhealthy fats, leading to meals with a high glycemic count. Sit-down restaurants, on the other hand, often have wider menu options, including salads, grilled proteins, and whole grain dishes, which align better with a low glycemic diet.

If possible, try to plan ahead. Look at the restaurant's menu online before you go. This way, you can take your time to analyze the options and decide on a low-glycemic meal without feeling rushed.

Moreover, don't hesitate to ask your server about the dish's preparation. Most restaurants are accommodating and willing to modify dishes to meet dietary needs. Requesting for dressings or sauces on the side, opting for steamed or grilled options instead of fried, or swapping out a side of potatoes for a salad, are just a few modifications that can help keep your meal within the low-glycemic range.

Remember, the goal is not to isolate yourself from social situations involving food but to navigate them in a way that aligns with your new dietary lifestyle. With a little planning and smart choices, you can enjoy dining out while maintaining your Low Glycemic Diet.

Conclusion

Congratulations on reaching the end of this comprehensive guide to the Low Glycemic Index (GI) Diet. Your determination to understand this health-promoting dietary approach is admirable.

Navigating through the intricacies of the Low GI Diet may have felt like a challenging task, but remember, each stride toward a healthier lifestyle is a triumph in its own right. The dedication you've shown by reading this far speaks volumes about your commitment to personal wellness.

So, what's the big takeaway from this guide? The Low Glycemic Index Diet isn't a fleeting trend. It's a scientifically grounded lifestyle shift that involves consuming foods that have a lesser effect on your blood sugar levels. This method not only aids in maintaining steady energy levels throughout the day but also contributes to weight management and overall health.

One of the most enticing aspects of the Low GI Diet is its flexibility. There's no call for extreme changes or complete elimination of food groups. Rather, it's about making smarter choices - opting for low-GI alternatives instead of high-GI foods. From whole grains to fresh fruits and vegetables, there's an expansive array of tasty and nutritious foods ready to be incorporated into your meals.

Initiating any new diet can seem intimidating, but remember, the initial step is often the toughest. Changes won't occur instantaneously, and that's perfectly fine. It's the persistent efforts and minor victories that accumulate over time. Be gentle with yourself and celebrate every accomplishment, irrespective of its size.

Whenever you feel swamped, recall why you embarked on this journey: to enhance your health and well-being. Keep this goal at the forefront as you navigate your path with the Low GI Diet. It's not about attaining perfection but about progression and making healthier choices one meal at a time.

As you proceed on your journey, don't hesitate to experiment with various low-G foods and recipes. Discover what suits you and your lifestyle best. After all, the most sustainable diet is the one that brings you joy and integrates effortlessly into your daily life.

In conclusion, we want to applaud you for taking the initiative to educate yourself on the Low Glycemic Index Diet. Your commitment to learning is the initial step towards transformation, and we're thrilled to see where this journey leads you. Remember, every step forward, no matter how small, is progress.

We hope this guide has offered valuable insights and practical advice to help you embark on or continue your journey with the Low GI Diet. Remember, the road to better health isn't a sprint; it's a marathon. So, keep moving forward, stay optimistic, and have faith in your ability to make healthier choices.

FAQs

What is a Low Glycemic Index Diet?

A Low Glycemic Index (GI) Diet involves consuming foods that have a lesser impact on blood sugar levels. The GI measures how a carbohydrate-containing food raises blood glucose. Foods are ranked based on how they compare to a reference standard - usually glucose or white bread.

What are the benefits of a Low GI Diet?

A Low GI Diet helps maintain balanced energy levels throughout the day, aids in weight management, and promotes overall health. It can also reduce your risk of developing type 2 diabetes and heart disease.

Can I eat any low-GI food in unlimited amounts on this diet?

No, portion control is still important when following a Low GI Diet. While these foods may not spike your blood sugar levels as much as high GI foods, consuming them in large quantities can still lead to weight gain and other health issues.

Does a Low GI Diet mean I have to eliminate certain food groups?

No, the Low GI Diet does not require you to eliminate any food groups. Instead, it encourages you to make smarter choices by opting for low-GI alternatives instead of high-GI foods.

How can I identify low-GI foods?

Low GI foods typically include whole grains, non-starchy vegetables, some fruits, and legumes. You can usually find GI values for different foods online or in a GI index book.

What if I feel overwhelmed while following the Low GI Diet?

It's normal to feel overwhelmed when starting a new diet. Remember, it's not about achieving perfection but rather about progress and making healthier choices one meal at a time. Be patient with yourself and celebrate every achievement.

Are there any risks associated with a Low GI Diet?

Generally, a Low GI Diet is considered safe for most people. However, it's always best to consult with a healthcare professional before starting any new diet. They can provide personalized advice based on your specific health needs and goals.

References and Helpful Links

Harvard Health. (2014, February 15). 8 principles of low-glycemic eating. https://www.health.harvard.edu/healthbeat/8-principles-of-low-glycemic-eating

Department of Health & Human Services. (n.d.). Carbohydrates and the glycaemic index. Better Health Channel. https://www.betterhealth.vic.gov.au/health/healthyliving/carbohydrates-and-the-glycaemic-index

Mph, S. C. M. (2022, February 25). Difference between glycemic index and glycemic load. Verywell Health. https://www.verywellhealth.com/glycemic-index-vs-load-5214363

Richards, L. (2021, February 8). What are high and low glycemic index foods? https://www.medicalnewstoday.com/articles/high-glycemic-index-foods

Watts, M. (2023, October 29). *Glycemic Index and diabetes - GI diet, GI foods & Benefits of low GI*. Diabetes. https://www.diabetes.co.uk/diet/glycaemic-index-diet-and-diabetes.html

Rd, R. a. M. (2023, October 27). Glycemic Index: What it is and how to use it. Healthline. https://www.healthline.com/nutrition/glycemic-index

Apd, D. C. (2023, February 24). *A beginner's guide to the low glycemic diet*. Healthline. https://www.healthline.com/nutrition/low-glycemic-diet#:~:text=Studies%20have%20shown%20that%20the,to%20reflect%20foods'%20overall%20healthiness.

Made in the USA
Monee, IL
06 October 2025